You can return this item to any library but please
note that not all libraries are open every day.
Items must be returned on or before the due date.
Failure to do so will result in overdue charges.
Items may be renewed unless requested by
another customer, in person or by telephone, on
two occasions only. Your membership card number
will be required.
Please look after this item – you may be charged
for any damage.

Headquarters:
Information, Culture & Community Learning,
Town Hall, Bournemouth BH2 6DY

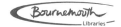

THIS IS A CARLTON BOOK

Text, illustrations and design copyright © 2008
Carlton Books Limited

This edition published by
Carlton Books Limited 2008
20 Mortimer Street
London W1T 3JW

A CIP catalogue record for this book is available from the British
Library.

ISBN 978-1-84732-069-8

Printed and bound in Singapore

Senior Executive Editor: Lisa Dyer
Senior Art Editor: Gulen Shevki-Taylor
Designer: Emma Wicks
Copy Editor: Jane Donovan
Production: Kate Pimm

Your **Carbon Footprint** is the amount of carbon dioxide emitted
due to your daily activities – from washing a load of laundry to
driving to work. See www.carbonfootprint.com for ways to reduce
your impact on the environment.

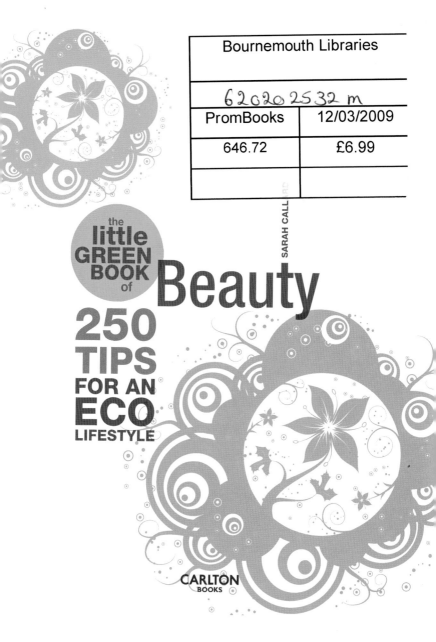

SARAH CALLARD

the little GREEN BOOK of Beauty

250 TIPS FOR AN ECO LIFESTYLE

CARLTON BOOKS

From coal tar in hair dyes to formaldehyde in nail varnishes, the average woman is exposed to as many as 175 chemicals from her beauty products every day that can cause conditions as mild as skin irritation or as serious as cancer.

It's not just the toxins in beauty products that are bad for the health either; synthetic chemicals from these products find their way from your home into waterways and soil, contaminating food and water supplies for all living things. The following tips highlight the environmental and health problems associated with lots of ingredients commonly found in beauty and bodycare products to help you make well-informed choices that are good for you and the planet.

1 HAVE A CLEAR OUT

Take a look at your bathroom cabinet and clear out everything but the essentials. If you've got more than one of any particular cosmetic product, pass it on, get rid of it and try not to buy duplicate products in the future.

2 STICK TO THE SHELF-LIFE

Bear in mind that natural products won't contain the same levels of chemical preservatives as other brands, so their shelf life will be shorter. Always use products before their 'best before' date and dispose of any after this time.

3 LOOK OUT FOR LABELS

Some labels such as 'hypoallergenic' don't have to be substantiated. Other labels such as 'unscented' or 'fragrance-free' don't ensure that the product doesn't contain fragrance, just that they have been used to mask the odour of other chemicals.

4 LOOK AT THE LABEL

Many of us are used to scanning food labels to check out salt and fat content and it is worth doing the same with cosmetics and beauty products. Lack of regulation means that literally hundreds of chemicals can be included in just one ingredient name – such as 'fragrance'.

5 WISE UP

Most people think that ingredients in personal care and cosmetic products are safety tested before they are sold but there is no such requirement under federal law in the US. Ingredients including mercury, lead and even placenta have found their way into cosmetics.

6 BE CAREFUL IF YOU'RE BREASTFEEDING

It pays to be extra cautious about the beauty products you use if you are breastfeeding. Studies have found that some chemicals, including a group of perfume chemicals still widely used in cosmetics, are stored in the mother's body fat and passed on to babies when they are breastfed.

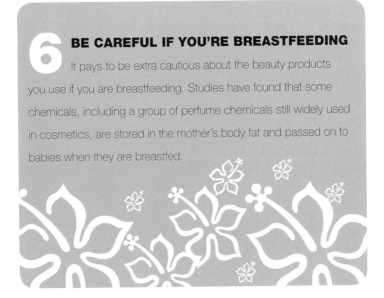

7

TOXINS IN BREAST MILK

A Swedish study revealed that triclosan, an ingredient found in products such as mouthwash, toothpaste and soap, has been found in high levels in 60% of human breast milk samples. Pregnant and nursing mothers should pay special attention to avoid using these products.

NOT JUST SKIN DEEP

The outer layer of our skin can be penetrated quite well by some oils, which are often used in products to carry the active ingredients into the deeper layers of the skin. Therefore, it makes sense to give more consideration to the products that you apply and leave on the skin.

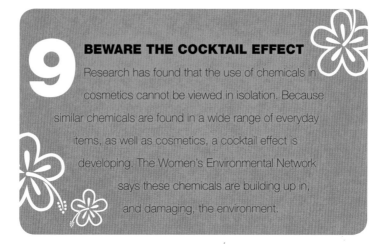

9 BEWARE THE COCKTAIL EFFECT

Research has found that the use of chemicals in cosmetics cannot be viewed in isolation. Because similar chemicals are found in a wide range of everyday items, as well as cosmetics, a cocktail effect is developing. The Women's Environmental Network says these chemicals are building up in, and damaging, the environment.

10 CHOOSE NATURAL TO AVOID HARMFUL TOXINS

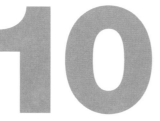

We absorb around 60% of what we put on our skin and the average woman comes into contact with as many as 175 different chemicals from the beauty products she uses every day. Choose natural products without synthetic or man-made ingredients to avoid the toxins.

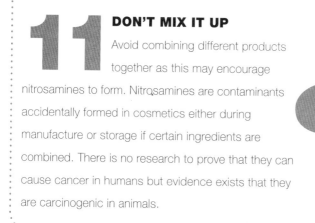

11 DON'T MIX IT UP

Avoid combining different products together as this may encourage nitrosamines to form. Nitrosamines are contaminants accidentally formed in cosmetics either during manufacture or storage if certain ingredients are combined. There is no research to prove that they can cause cancer in humans but evidence exists that they are carcinogenic in animals.

12 BE CHEMICALLY-AWARE

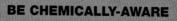

The National Institute of Occupational Safety and Health in the US lists 884 chemicals in use by the cosmetic industry as toxic substances, including phthalates, acrylamide, formaldehyde and even some pesticides. Many of them have been linked to health scares including cancer and gender disruption. Reduce the number of products you use to avoid overexposure to the chemicals found in cosmetics.

13 SHOW YOUR SENSITIVE SIDE

Around 40% of the British population is now affected by allergies and, according to Allergy UK, over-exposure to chemicals can trigger a sensitivity that may lead to an allergy such as asthma, eczema or hay fever. Choosing natural products will reduce your exposure to chemicals.

14 CHOOSE TO BE FRAGRANCE-FREE

Manufacturers are not legally required to list any of the potentially hundreds of chemicals in a single product's fragrance mixture. Fragrances can contain neurotoxins and are known allergens. Avoid them by choosing products fragranced only with pure essential oils.

15 SNIFF AROUND

Although it does have to be listed in the ingredients, fragrance in a product can appear in a variety of different ways so it's good to familiarize yourself with the different terms. Perfume, parfum, aroma and fragrance are all common words used for perfume in a product.

16 COMMON SCENTS

Look out for the word 'fragrance' on ingredients lists. Current legislation doesn't restrict the quantities or combinations of fragrance chemicals that can be used in everyday cosmetics. This means that it's not unusual for some products to contain as much as between 50 and 100 fragrances.

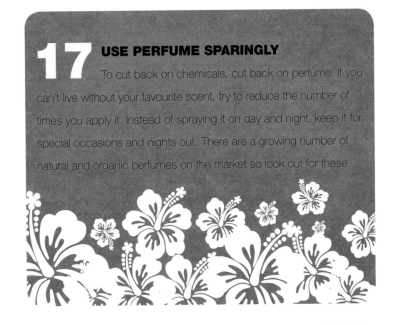

17 USE PERFUME SPARINGLY

To cut back on chemicals, cut back on perfume. If you can't live without your favourite scent, try to reduce the number of times you apply it. Instead of spraying it on day and night, keep it for special occasions and nights out. There are a growing number of natural and organic perfumes on the market so look out for these.

18 ORGANIC SCENTS

Avoid the synthetic fragrances that may contain hormone-disrupting chemicals such as phthalates and opt for organic fragrances instead. There are plenty of wonderful, certified organic scents to choose from and brands to look out for include: Organic Apoteke, Aveda and Parseme.

19

AVOID MUSK FOR DEERS' SAKE

Many upmarket perfumes contain substances such as musk and civet. Musk comes from the gland of a male musk deer which has been hunted to near extinction. Civet is a secretion from civet cats and there are reports that they are tormented to increase the secretions they produce. Avoid fragrances containing these ingredients.

20

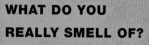

WHAT DO YOU REALLY SMELL OF?

Other unsavoury ingredients commonly found in perfumes and fragrances include castorium and ambergris. Castorium comes from beavers, which are reportedly trapped and killed before the secretion is obtained from the beavers' genital glands, and ambergris comes from the intestines of sperm whales. Many marine mammal protection laws ban trade in ambergris.

21 AVOIDING SLS

Sodium lauryl sulphate (SLS) is a known irritant and a common ingredient in many beauty and bodycare products. Found in most shampoos, hair conditioners, body washes and bubble baths, SLS is a strong detergent and foaming agent. It can irritate eyes, skin and mucous membranes and has been linked to allergic reactions.

22 CHOOSE SLES RATHER THAN SLS

Sodium laurel sulphate (SLS) is a known irritant (see tip 21 above), but sodium lauryl ethyl sulphate (SLES) is a much milder foaming agent derived from coconut, which is thought to be much gentler on the skin. If you are using commercial, non-organic products, choose one with SLES instead of SLS.

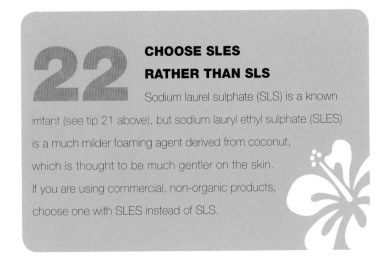

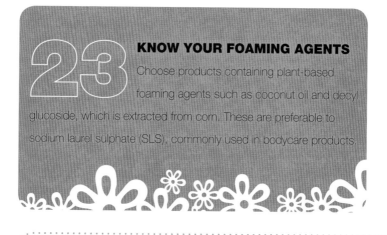

KNOW YOUR FOAMING AGENTS

Choose products containing plant-based foaming agents such as coconut oil and decyl glucoside, which is extracted from corn. These are preferable to sodium laurel sulphate (SLS), commonly used in bodycare products.

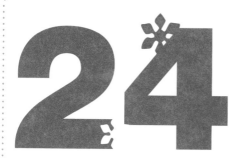

CHECK PRODUCTS FOR SODIUM BENZOATE

A common preservative in cosmetics and food is sodium benzoate, an antimicrobial preservative. However, it has been linked to health problems including gastric irritation, numbing of the mouth and nettle rash. It is widely used in products such as cosmetic wipes, where the chemicals are likely to remain on the skin, so avoid it if possible.

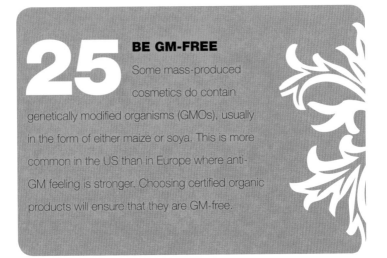

25 BE GM-FREE

Some mass-produced cosmetics do contain genetically modified organisms (GMOs), usually in the form of either maize or soya. This is more common in the US than in Europe where anti-GM feeling is stronger. Choosing certified organic products will ensure that they are GM-free.

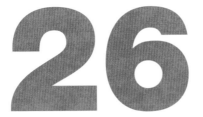

26 READ BETWEEN THE LINES

Watch out for gender-bending chemicals known as phthalates which are often hidden in the catchall phrase of 'fragrance' on beauty and bodycare products. They have been identified as hormone disrupters and studies have found they have reduced the male hormone action in rats.

27 BE CAREFUL WHAT YOU WASH DOWN YOUR SINK

Triclosan, a common ingredient in toothpaste, deodorant and soap, is known to be environmentally harmful. It can be converted to cancer-causing dioxin when exposed to sunlight in water and has been classified as toxic to aquatic organisms and the aquatic environment.

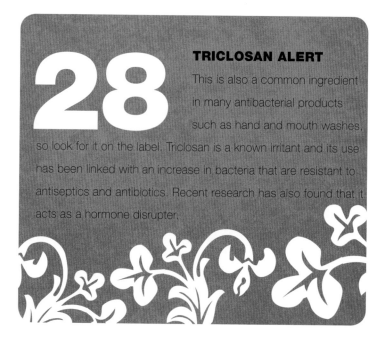

28 TRICLOSAN ALERT

This is also a common ingredient in many antibacterial products such as hand and mouth washes, so look for it on the label. Triclosan is a known irritant and its use has been linked with an increase in bacteria that are resistant to antiseptics and antibiotics. Recent research has also found that it acts as a hormone disrupter.

29

DON'T PEG IT!

Propylene glycol is a wetting agent and solvent used in shampoos, deodorants and aftershave, among others. It is also one of the main ingredients in antifreeze and brake fluid. Polyethylene glycol, which often appears as PEG, is used to dissolve grease and is found in lots of facial cleansers as well as oven cleaners.

30

SAY NO TO NANOPARTICLES

Nanoparticles are one of the latest buzzwords in the beauty world and they are already being used in a wide range of products, from lipsticks to foundations. Manufacturers don't have to list them in the ingredients, however, so they are hard to avoid but worth doing so because there are concerns that nanoparticles can end up in the bloodstream and cause inflammation.

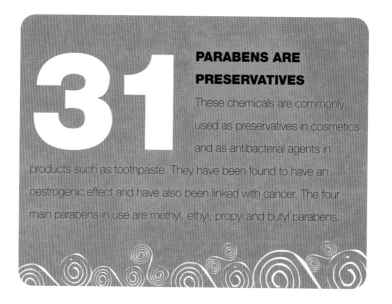

31

PARABENS ARE PRESERVATIVES

These chemicals are commonly used as preservatives in cosmetics and as antibacterial agents in products such as toothpaste. They have been found to have an oestrogenic effect and have also been linked with cancer. The four main parabens in use are methyl, ethyl, propyl and butyl parabens.

32

PACK IN THE PETROLEUM PRODUCTS

Petroleum-based ingredients such as petrolatum, which is also known as baby oil, strips the natural oils from the skin, causing chapping and dryness, and even premature ageing. The manufacture of petroleum-based ingredients also has a major impact on the environment.

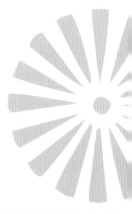

33 AVOID PHTHALATES

Phthalates are a family of chemicals often used to soften plastics. They were banned from children's toys after it was discovered they were ingesting the chemical by sucking. Phthalates are still used in a number of products, such as hairspray, deodorants, body lotions, fragrances and nail polishes, usually to soften the formula or make it more flexible. However, the fact remains that they have been linked with birth defects and reproductive health problems.

34 CHOOSE PRODUCTS WITH FEWER INGREDIENTS

The more natural a product, the fewer ingredients it is likely to have. A good clue that a product is full of chemicals is the length of the ingredients list, so if in doubt avoid it. The more ingredients it contains, the more likely it is that you may react badly to one of them.

35

SEEK OUT FREEZE-DRIED HERBAL INGREDIENTS

Parabens are often added to beauty products to preserve them but there are concerns about their safety. As an alternative, some manufacturers are moving towards using freeze-dried herbal ingredients, which don't need to be preserved.

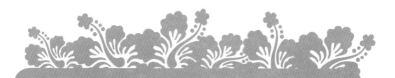

36

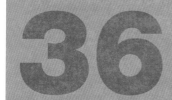

HIGH IN HERBS

Herbs such as aloe vera and lavender have been traditionally used for their cleansing, moisturizing and soothing qualities. Products high in herbal content rather than synthetics are not only natural but also very effective. Look for organic or wild-crafted herbal products to ensure the environment is also being protected.

37 BEWARE OF EMPTY CLAIMS

The cosmetic industry loves to bandy around words such as 'organic' and 'natural' but without certification they are meaningless. This is because, legally, a product containing as little as 1% of natural ingredients can call itself a natural product.

38 WHAT IS A NATURAL INGREDIENT?

A natural substance is any plant or animal extract, or any rock or mineral obtained from the earth. It is possible to make exact copies of natural substances using raw materials from coal tar and petroleum and many manufacturers choose to synthesize ingredients rather than to extract them from natural sources.

39 NATURAL PRODUCTS HAVE A SHORTER SHELF-LIFE

Be aware that many natural products have a shorter shelf-life than conventional products because they don't use as many preservatives. Don't use products beyond their 'best before' date. If there isn't a date listed on the product it will have been formulated to have a minimum shelf-life of 30 months, so discard it after this period.

40 CHOOSE TO USE PLANT RATHER THAN MINERAL OILS

Mineral oils are derived from petrochemicals and are therefore not sustainable. As well as being environmentally unsound they have also been linked to allergic reactions when applied to the skin. Plant oils such as olive and almond oil contain essential fatty acids, vitamins and other nutrients which nourish the skin naturally.

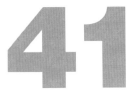

KNOWING IT'S NATURAL

One way to be sure that a European product is as natural as it claims to be is if it has been certified by the BDIH in Germany. This means the ingredients have to be from a plant or mineral source; most petroleum-based and synthetic ingredients are not permitted, and neither are GM ingredients.

SMELLS GOOD NATURALLY

Products containing natural fragrances are the most environmentally friendly choice. Fragrance from herbal infusions, floral waters and essential oils using organic herbs and spring water are the gentle way to smell good without the use of synthetic chemicals.

43
GO FOR PRODUCTS WITH PLANT-BASED INGREDIENTS

Natural, plant-based ingredients are the best option for any products that are likely to be absorbed into your skin. Pure essential oils have a therapeutic effect without stripping the skin of its natural oils. If you are pregnant, however, check with your doctor first about which oils are safe to use.

44
USE ESSENTIAL OILS

Choose products containing organic essential oils as many of them have the added benefit of acting as natural preservatives. Make sure you store them away from sunlight, preferably in dark glass bottles, and that way they will last longer.

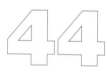

45

MORE THAN A LITTLE SENSITIVE

Even natural and organic products can cause allergic reactions on people with particularly sensitive skin. Essential oils and natural ingredients can be extremely potent so if you are at all concerned do a patch test on a small area of skin before slathering a new product all over your face or body.

46

BE CAUTIOUS WITH OILS

Although essential oils are by far the greener choice over synthesized versions, it still pays to be cautious when using them as some may cause allergic reactions among very sensitive users. The key oils to be cautious with are tea tree, eucalyptus and citrus-based oils.

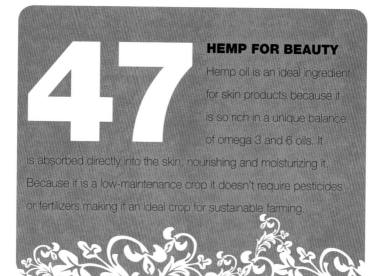

47

HEMP FOR BEAUTY

Hemp oil is an ideal ingredient for skin products because it is so rich in a unique balance of omega 3 and 6 oils. It is absorbed directly into the skin, nourishing and moisturizing it. Because it is a low-maintenance crop it doesn't require pesticides or fertilizers making it an ideal crop for sustainable farming.

48

CHOOSE ESSENTIAL OILS, NOT SYNTHETIC FRAGRANCES

Manufacturers of synthetic fragrance oils do not have to disclose the ingredients used in their making, so you really have no idea what they contain although they are subject to safety guidelines. They are cheaper than essential oils though so are often used in beauty and bodycare products.

49

CHOOSE LOCAL AND HANDMADE

An increasing number of small manufacturers making handmade beauty care products using natural and organic ingredients. The production methods are usually small scale so have minimal environmental impact and local production also cuts down on carbon emissions caused by transportation.

50

COLD-BLENDED IS BEST

Some manufacturers, such as Paul Penders, are developing cold-blended cosmetics. Many conventional products are manufactured using heat-processing, which can destroy the bioactive ingredients. Cold-blending protects the ingredients, thereby making the final product more effective.

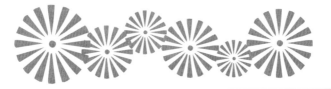

51 GOOD ENOUGH TO EAT

A current trend in the beauty world is for making cosmetics using food-grade ingredients such as fruit, oats and vegetables that are designed to nourish your skin from the outside in. British cosmetic company NOe (Natural Organic edible) and US company Be Fine Food Skincare are good examples of this trend. Their products are natural and preservative-free.

52 LOOK OUT FOR ORGANIC

The global market for organic cosmetics is growing and in 2006 1,600 organic products were launched worldwide. However, be cautious: manufacturers are not legally required to obtain organic certification to make organic claims. Make sure the products you buy carry the logos of either the Soil Association, Ecocert or USDA Organic (United States Department of Agriculture). These products contain ingredients that are assessed to be safe to human health and guarantee that their manufacture and use causes minimum environmental impact.

READ THE PACKAGING

Many cosmetic and skincare products contain ingredients classified as food items. In the UK look out for letters UKROFS followed by a number on the label, which shows that the product has been approved by the United Kingdom Register of Organic Food Standards.

GO ORGANIC

By using certified organic beauty products you will ensure you are not coming into contact with synthetic fragrances and colours. Different certifiers have different organic standards so it's worth checking who allows what ingredients. The Soil Association, for example, doesn't permit the use of the foaming agent sodium laurel sulphate (SLS), solvents or parabens.

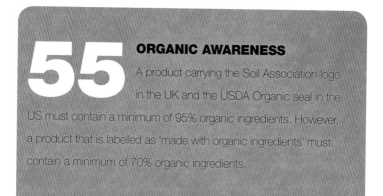

55 ORGANIC AWARENESS

A product carrying the Soil Association logo in the UK and the USDA Organic seal in the US must contain a minimum of 95% organic ingredients. However, a product that is labelled as 'made with organic ingredients' must contain a minimum of 70% organic ingredients.

56 BUY ORGANIC FOR SKIN ALLERGIES

People who suffer from sensitive skin and skin allergies sometimes find that using organic products is less likely to cause a reaction. Allergy sufferers can sometimes tolerate organic products better because they only contain tiny amounts of synthetic chemicals.

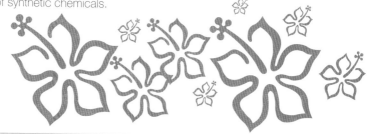

57 GO BIODYNAMIC

There are an increasing number of biodynamic beautycare products on the market. These are products made using ingredients that have been produced using biodynamic methods. Biodynamic farming is sometimes seen as the next step up from organic farming. Brands to look out for include Dr Hauschka and Jurlique.

58 LOOK FOR THE LEAPING BUNNY

Products with the leaping bunny logo mean that the product has been approved under the international Humane Cosmetics Standard (www.eceae.org) and guarantees that the product itself – or any of the ingredients it contains – have not been tested on animals. The organization, a coalition of animal-protection groups from the European Union and North America, is the world's only international criteria for cosmetic or toiletry products that are 'Not Tested on Animals'. See also www.leapingbunny.org.

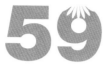

59 ETHICAL BEAUTY

Manufacturers, by law, have to test their products and it is up to them how they do it, so use your purchasing power to send a message to cosmetics companies that testing on animals is unacceptable. The European Union has passed a ban on animal testing in cosmetics, starting in 2009 with a complete ban in 2013.

60 CHECK IF YOUR BRAND IS CRUELTY-FREE

Several anti-vivisection websites feature search engines that allow you to see if your favourite brand has been approved under the Humane Cosmetics Standard. This includes European and North American manufacturers such as the American Anti-vivisection Society (www.aavs.org) and the British Union for the Abolition of Vivisection (www.buav.org).

61 DON'T BE FOOLED BY THE BAN

Despite the fact that there is a UK ban on cosmetic testing on animals, this doesn't necessarily mean that British cosmetics companies are cruelty-free. Many leading brands are still using products and ingredients that have been manufactured and tested overseas.

62 AVOID PALM-OIL PRODUCTS

Unethical sourcing of palm oil for cosmetics and a wide range of other products is having a devastating effect on the environment, endangered species and indigenous populations around the world according to the World Wildlife Fund (WWF). The Body Shop is the first global cosmetics company to introduce sustainable palm oil into its product lines.

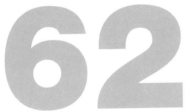

63 BUY FAIRTRADE COTTON WOOL

Make sure that your cotton wool isn't being produced at the expense of the workers creating it by buying fairtrade-certified cotton wool and cotton buds (swabs). Look for the International Fairtrade Association FTO mark on products (see www.ifat.org). In the UK fairtrade products must be registered by the Fairtrade Foundation and carry the fairtrade mark (see www.fairtrade.org.uk).

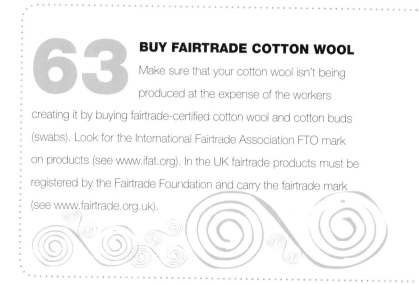

64 CHOOSE ETHICAL BEAUTY

Following the international success of the fairtrade food market, ethical beauty and bodycare products are moving in the same direction. Knowing that the product has been made without harming the workers or the environment is becoming more important and some brands are using ethically sourced ingredients such as sustainably harvested herbs.

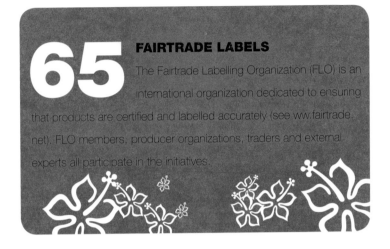

65 FAIRTRADE LABELS

The Fairtrade Labelling Organization (FLO) is an international organization dedicated to ensuring that products are certified and labelled accurately (see ww.fairtrade.net). FLO members; producer organizations, traders and external experts all participate in the initiatives.

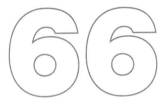

66 DON'T BELIEVE THE HYPE

Avoid getting sucked into the advertising hype. Manufacturers employ marketing techniques to exploit women's insecurities about their body image, often using enhanced images of men and women to sell products. Studies in the US found that 70% of women say they feel worse about their own looks after reading women's magazines, so view advertisements and magazine pages with a degree of healthy cynicism.

67 BUY FROM YOUR LOCAL HEALTH FOOD STORE

Visit your local health food or organic store when you are buying beauty products and cosmetics. They will be more knowledgeable than staff in supermarkets and larger stores and will be able to advise you on the right sort of product for your skin.

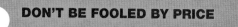

68 DON'T BE FOOLED BY PRICE

Some of the more expensive products are not necessarily better than cheaper versions. Products claiming added active ingredients are often pricier than more basic products but beware – the active ingredients may not transfer effectively from the laboratory to the final product.

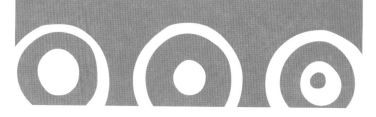

69 BEWARE OF 'NEW, IMPROVED' PRODUCTS

The average market life of a beauty product is between two and three years and so manufacturers have to be constantly coming up with new ways to market products. Be aware that these new formulations are often just a way to boost sales and sometimes the only new thing is the name.

70 SUPPLEMENT YOUR REGIME

There is a wide range of vitamin and mineral supplements available specifically to boost hair, skin and nails. Combination formulas, such as Viridian's Beauty Complex, provide a one-stop shop for women wanting to boost their general appearance. Individual supplements can be taken for specific areas, such as silica for hair and nails and omega-3 fatty acids for skin.

71 CHANGE YOUR DIET

Following a diet high in antioxidants such as vitamins C and E will boost your looks and improve your immune system at the same time. Avoiding foods high in saturated fats and eating a diet based on fruit and vegetables are two of the best ways to preserve your looks and protect your skin from ageing and pollution.

72 A NATURAL BEAUTY FIX-IT

Making sure you have enough sleep – generally eight hours – will boost the appearance of your skin. This is because it gives your body the chance to repair and regenerate tissue. It is also important to get enough exercise which helps to boost circulation and stimulate skin cleansing.

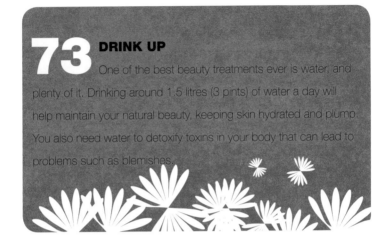

73 DRINK UP

One of the best beauty treatments ever is water, and plenty of it. Drinking around 1.5 litres (3 pints) of water a day will help maintain your natural beauty, keeping skin hydrated and plump. You also need water to detoxify toxins in your body that can lead to problems such as blemishes.

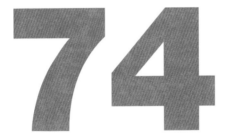

74 KEEP HYDRATED WITHOUT THE WASTE

Drinking enough water is essential for optimum health and beauty but buying bottles of mineral water is not a good environmental option due to the amount of waste. Drinking tap water is the greenest option – you can elminate added chlorine by using a water filter.

75

EAT STRAWBERRIES

High in antioxidants, strawberries can be beneficial in the fight against premature ageing and wrinkles. They are particularly high in vitamin C, which is important for the formation of collagen – a key element that helps to keep skin firm. Strawberries also help to protect against broken capillaries beneath the skin's surface.

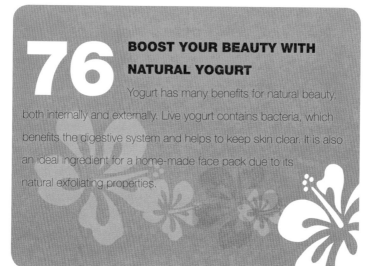

76

BOOST YOUR BEAUTY WITH NATURAL YOGURT

Yogurt has many benefits for natural beauty, both internally and externally. Live yogurt contains bacteria, which benefits the digestive system and helps to keep skin clear. It is also an ideal ingredient for a home-made face pack due to its natural exfoliating properties.

77

CHOOSE GOAT'S MILK

Goat's milk helps to seal moisture into the skin and maintain its natural pH level, making it an ideal ingredient for soap. In addition, goat's milk is higher in fat and richer than cow's milk so is extremely moisturizing. It also naturally contains alpha-hydroxy acids which are known for their rejuvenating qualities.

78

DRINK GREEN TEA

Favoured by celebrities including Sophie Dahl and Victoria Beckham, green tea has a number of beauty benefits. It is naturally rich in antioxidants, which help to protect against free radicals and premature ageing. The leaves can also be used as a gentle exfoliant to give your skin a healthy glow.

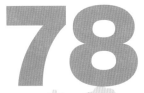

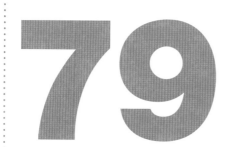

DETOX TWICE A YEAR

One way to get clearer eyes and a radiant glow is to detoxify. Natural health experts recommend detoxing twice a year – around spring and autumn – to give your skin and overall health a boost. Ridding your body of everyday toxins can help to improve the texture and appearance of your skin and hair.

80 LOOK TO THE EAST

For centuries Ayurvedic medicine has been using herbal remedies to treat skin complaints. Companies such as Pukka Herbs (www.pukkaherbs.com) have created Ayurvedic formulations designed to soothe irritated and inflamed skin, and to boost its general appearance. Pukka's Cleanse Tea is a blend of herbs designed to boost radiant skin.

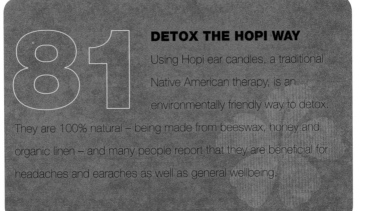

DETOX THE HOPI WAY

81 Using Hopi ear candles, a traditional Native American therapy, is an environmentally friendly way to detox. They are 100% natural – being made from beeswax, honey and organic linen – and many people report that they are beneficial for headaches and earaches as well as general wellbeing.

VISIT A HEALTH SPA

82 For an indulgent but natural treat, visit a spa. Treatments such as massages, facials and hot stone treatments all help the body to relax and detoxify naturally. Make sure the spa you visit uses organic or at least natural products during its therapies.

83 SPEND TIME ON YOURSELF

Time and energy put into making your own home beauty treatments from natural ingredients should be considered part of a pampering programme, rather than another chore. Set aside time to make the beauty treatments yourself and enjoy the whole process. You will find it much more satisfying than spending lots of time and of money shopping in a busy store.

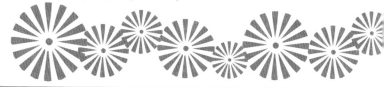

84 TRY HOT STONE THERAPY

Avoid lots of pills and potions and try hot stone therapy instead. This therapy has been used by different cultures for centuries to ease symptoms such as aches and strains, arthritis and even insomnia. Warm stone expands the blood vessels, allowing blood to move faster round the body.

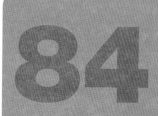

85

A MARBLE MASSAGE

A great way to soothe sore feet is to give them a marble massage. Add a layer of marbles to a foot bath containing a few drops of essential oil and roll your feet around on them while you soak.

86

STAY BEAUTIFUL WITH A DAILY DOSE OF YOGA

Daily yoga can help to improve your appearance naturally. Practised regularly, breathing and stretching exercises can reduce the appearance of wrinkles, dark circles under the eyes and bring colour to your cheeks. It will also improve your overall health and fitness.

87

HAVE A MASSAGE

A relaxing massage has physical as well as psychological benefits. Massage helps to improve skin colour and tone by removing dead skin cells and boosting circulation. It aids detoxification and encourages more efficient waste removal, and can encourage better lymph drainage and so reduce swelling.

88

EXERCISE YOUR FACE MUSCLES

Completing a regular session of face and neck muscles can help improve the elasticity and appearance of the skin. Regular stretching exercises help to boost circulation and tone up the muscles around the eyes, necks and cheeks without the need for any products.

89 BE A HONEY MONSTER

Manuka honey is one of the best ingredients to incorporate into your natural beauty regime. It has natural moisturizing, nourishing, healing and rejuvenating properties as well as being a natural humectant (a substance that attracts and preserves moisture). Manuka honey can be applied topically and appears in a wide range of beauty products.

90 NOURISH SKIN WITH AVOCADO

Avocado is arguably the most important food for well-nourished skin. It provides essential fats necessary to prevent wrinkles and dryness. Incorporate avocado into your diet on a regular basis and apply it, mixed with natural yogurt, once a week as a face pack to get the benefits, internally and externally.

91 SOLVE PROBLEM AREAS WITH LEMON

Dry and discoloured skin on knees and elbows can be dealt with by using a fresh lemon. Cut it in half and sprinkle with a teaspoon of sugar, then rub the lemon halves into elbows and knees for a few minutes.

92 CLEAR SKIN WITH STEAM

This is particularly good for oily and blemished skin. Bring a pot of water with fresh herbs such as parsley and peppermint to the boil, remove from the heat and stand for a few minutes. Put a towel over your head and lean over the infusion for ten minutes.

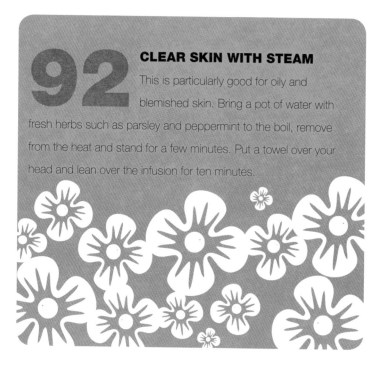

93

LOOK FOR PURE FACE MASKS

If you do choose a commercial face mask, look for one that is hypo-allergenic and free from perfume, parabens or colours. If you make your own from all-natural ingredients use distilled water instead of ordinary tap water, which can be high in minerals and may irritate sensitive skins.

94

GET A FACELIFT WITH EGG WHITE

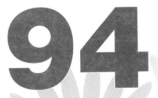

Egg whites can be used to give an instant, natural facelift. Dab the whites directly onto lined areas and allow to dry before continuing your usual beauty routine. This gives skin an instant lift and helps to reduce the appearance of wrinkles. Egg whites can also be combined with honey and lemon juice for a reviving face pack.

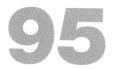

95 A TASTE OF HONEY

Honey is well known for its antibacterial properties and ability to heal wounds, as well as its skin moisturizing and nourishing benefits. A natural humectant, it draws water to the skin. Mixed with olive oil and brown sugar it makes an effective skin exfoliant. It can also be used as a face mask, or with olive oil as a hair mask.

96 YOGURT IS A NATURAL BEAUTY TREATMENT

Natural yogurt, ideally organic, can be used to reduce redness and irritation on skin. It can also be applied to the face like a face pack due to its cleansing and moisturizing properties. Natural yogurt is particularly beneficial for sunburn and acts as an effective aftersun.

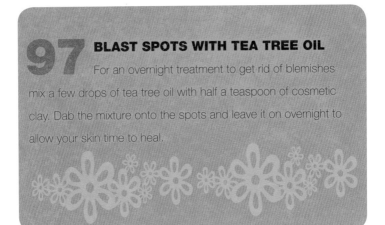

97 BLAST SPOTS WITH TEA TREE OIL

For an overnight treatment to get rid of blemishes mix a few drops of tea tree oil with half a teaspoon of cosmetic clay. Dab the mixture onto the spots and leave it on overnight to allow your skin time to heal.

98 ZAP SPOTS WITH HONEY

Honey contains phytochemicals that have powerful anti-inflammatory and antimicrobial properties. It is increasingly used to treat skin disorders because it speeds up healing and alleviates infection. These qualities also makes it a great treatment for getting rid of blemishes. Dab some honey onto an affected area at bedtime and you'll soon see the difference.

99

IMPROVE YOUR SKIN WITH GARLIC

Garlic has many health-giving properties such as improving circulation and enhancing the flow of nutrients and oxygen around the body. It also boasts the antifungal chemical allicin and contains compounds that help the body to detoxify. This makes it ideal for people prone to spots.

100

HOMEOPATHY FOR HEALTHY SKIN

Homeopathy works by treating like with like. Tiny amounts of the remedies which are made from plant, animal or mineral extracts are used to treat symptoms and it is a very safe type of treatment. Homeopathy can be used to treat various skin problems including acne, eczema and allergic reactions.

101

MOISTURIZER IS KEY

The vast majority of women, and an increasing number of men, think that moisturizer is one of the key beauty products in the fight against ageing and wrinkles, and around 92% of women use a moisturizer every day. Make sure yours is as natural as possible to reduce your exposure to chemicals.

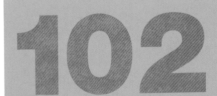

102

COMBAT DRY SKIN WITH EFAS

Essential fatty acids (EFAs) are crucial for our overall health. They can also play a role in natural skincare. Some of the first signs of EFA deficiency are dry, flaky skin, dull hair and brittle nails. Make sure your diet is high in oily fish, nuts and seeds, and consider supplementing with EFA capsules.

103 MOISTURIZE WITH OLIVE OIL

For dry skin use olive oil, organic if possible. It has excellent moisturizing properties and has been traditionally used as an intensive conditioning and moisturizing treatment for areas prone to dry skin such as elbows, knees and feet. For great results, apply at night for smoother skin when you wake up.

104 GET YOUR ANTIOXIDANTS NATURALLY

Antioxidants are one of the key weapons in the battle against wrinkles and ageing skin. These days, many mainstream products market themselves as high in antioxidants but it may be that a diet rich in fruit such as strawberries, which are an extremely good source of vitamin C, is a more effective way of boosting your antioxidant intake.

105

BE SCEPTICAL OF PRODUCTS WITH VITAMIN A

Studies have shown that vitamin A, or retinol, can help to reduce the appearance of wrinkles. However, the type of vitamin A found in beauty products is a very diluted form which is likely to be far less effective. This is because at high concentrations it can cause side effects such as peeling and stinging.

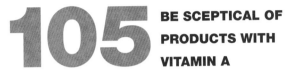

106

DO PEPTIDES REALLY PEP UP YOUR SKIN?

Peptides have recently been a buzzword in the beauty industry. They are thought to promote production of collagen, thereby, improving the elasticity and appearance of skin, making it look younger and healthier. However, boosting your diet with vitamin C-rich foods, which is crucial for the formation of collagen, is a more natural alternative.

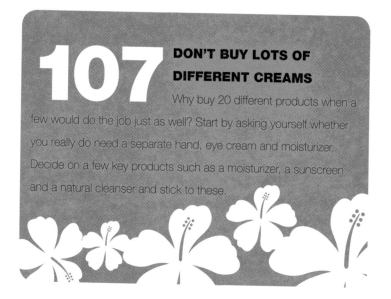

107 DON'T BUY LOTS OF DIFFERENT CREAMS

Why buy 20 different products when a few would do the job just as well? Start by asking yourself whether you really do need a separate hand, eye cream and moisturizer. Decide on a few key products such as a moisturizer, a sunscreen and a natural cleanser and stick to these.

108 THE NEW 'COSMECEUTICALS'

The term 'cosmeceutical' is used to describe cosmetic products that act like drugs in the way that they function on the skin. Although the market is growing rapidly research has revealed there isn't much difference between these and more basic products. Products typically labelled as cosmeceuticals include anti-ageing creams.

109

BETTER OFF WITHOUT BOTOX?

Botox is now seen as a mainstream beauty treatment, but is it safe? Common side effects include mild bruising and sometimes drooping of the eyebrow or eyelid. In high doses it can be toxic and cause serious health problems. Perhaps the best option is to avoid the sun and accept wrinkles as an inevitable part of growing old gracefully.

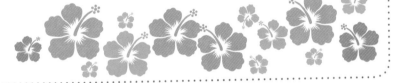

110

BLINDED BY SCIENCE

Products claiming to get rid of wrinkles overnight with the latest skin-boosting technology may sound impressive but probably won't live up to the hype. A simple, chemical-free beauty regime and healthy lifestyle may be just as effective.

111 AHAS MAY NOT PROVIDE THE RESULTS YOU WANT

The long term effects of alpha-hydroxy acids (AHAs), a common ingredient in cosmetics, are not yet known. One such chemical, salicylic acid, is banned in the EU from toiletries for use by children under the age of three, with the exception of shampoo.

112 KNOW YOUR AHAS

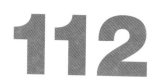

Alpha-hydroxy acids (AHAs) are used in products such as moisturizers and exfoliants. They effectively remove the outer layer of skin and are known for their anti-ageing effects. However, research has revealed concerns that they could cause increased sun-sensitivity and the risk of sun-related skin cancers.

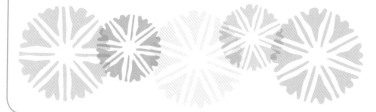

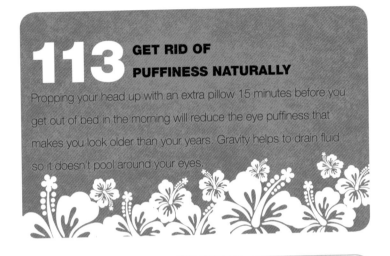

113 GET RID OF PUFFINESS NATURALLY

Propping your head up with an extra pillow 15 minutes before you get out of bed in the morning will reduce the eye puffiness that makes you look older than your years. Gravity helps to drain fluid so it doesn't pool around your eyes.

114 CHILL OUT

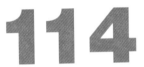

Cooling your eyelids can also help to eliminate puffiness naturally. Apply a cold tea bag and a slice of cucumber or potato to each eye, straight from the fridge, for 10 minutes to give your eyes a refreshing boost and deflate under-eye bags. Alternatively, keep an organic under-eye gel in the fridge and apply when needed for a tightening effect. Excess sodium or alcohol in the diet can also be factors in eye puffiness, so increase your water intake and eliminate toxins from your diet to help reduce puffy eyes.

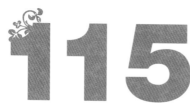

115

BE SUSPICIOUS OF ANTI-AGEING PRODUCTS

Like it or not, no product can prevent ageing, something worth remembering the next time you are tempted to shell out for the latest age-defying cream. Instead, make sure you drink lots of water, have enough essential fatty acids and a diet rich in fruit and vegetables.

116

ROSEHIP OIL FOR MATURE SKINS

Although no beauty product can ward off the signs of ageing, mature skin benefits from rose hip oil. This plant oil contains nutrients to keep skin soft and supple. It is also extremely beneficial for people with scars or stretchmarks and will help to reduce their appearance. However, make sure it has been ethically sourced.

117 COFFEE GETS RID OF CELLULITE

Used coffee grounds can be used as a body exfoliator to get rid of cellulite. Take the used grounds from your morning coffee and rub them onto problem areas such as thighs during your shower for a natural cellulite treatment.

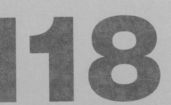

118 BEAT CELLULITE WITH SAGE

Sage is also known for its cellulite-busting properties so try to incorporate plenty of the fresh herb into your diet. It works by improving the digestion and breaking down the fatty deposits in the body which cause cellulite.

119 EXFOLIATE WITH CAUTION

Exfoliants, such as AHAs, are chemicals that soften or dissolve the outer layer of dead skin cells. They may well improve the appearance of fine lines, but they have also been known to cause skin damage and some people are extremely sensitive to them.

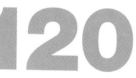

120 NATURALLY ROUGH

Use an organic cotton muslin face cloth as part of your skincare regime. As well as having less environmental impact than conventional cotton, organic muslins will also be better for your skin. They act as a very gentle natural exfoliant to remove dead skin cells without causing irritation.

121 GUARD AGAINST SUN DAMAGE

Despite an increase in the amount of sunscreen we are using, the rates of skin cancer continue to increase, which is not surprising as we are battling with greater pollution, ozone depletion, unregulated tanning salons and longer lifespans. One theory, though not proven, is that damage is enhanced by exposure to some of the ingredients used in sunscreens. In particular, avoid: parabens (butyl-, ethyl-, methyl- and propyl-), PABAs (para-aminobenzoic acid), padimate-O or parsol 1789, and benzophenone, homosalate or octy-methoxycinnamate (octinoxate).

122 CHOOSE YOUR SUNSCREEN CAREFULLY

A report by the Environmental Working Group (EWG) in the US revealed that 84% of 831 name-brand sunscreens offered inadequate protection from the sun or contain ingredients with significant safety concerns. Only 16% were considered safe and effective.

123 BEAUTY MINEFIELD

Titanium oxide, which is a common ingredient in many sunscreens, and talc have been linked to environmental damage during the mining process and manufacture. Avoid talc when possible because it has also been associated with health problems such as ovarian cancer.

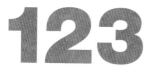

124 STAY OUT OF THE SUN

One of the most ageing things you can do to your skin is expose it to the sun, but if you have to be out in strong sunlight for prolonged periods, sunscreens are essential. There are an increasing number of natural sunscreens available but the best alternative is to wear a hat with a brim and stay out of the sun altogether, particularly in the middle of the day.

125 WATCH OUT FOR SUN SENSITIVITY

We are all much more aware of the need to protect ourselves from the UV rays of the sun, but some of the beauty products available actually increase sun sensitivity in certain people. This is true of products containing vitamin A, also known as retinol.

126 CHOOSE A BIODEGRADABLE 'BLOCK' SUNSCREEN

Sunscreens reduce the risk of skin cancer but they don't protect you from the sun's rays. Many contain chemicals that are not biodegradable but can wash off into the water supply, too. Most sunscreens offer a combination of both chemical and physical-barrier ingredients to protect you from the sun. Zinc oxide is the best physical-barrier screen as it has no harmful side-effects, no extra ingredients and is a mineral, so it is not absorbed into the bloodstream. Traditionally available in the thick white formula, there are now transparent versions.

127 AVOID USING A HIGH SPF WHEN YOU DON'T NEED IT

Remember you don't need a moisturizer with an added Sun Protection Factor overnight. Check that the products you are using don't have any added extra ingredients that you don't need in order to reduce your exposure to an unnecessary number of chemicals.

128 ALOE SOOTHES SUNBURN

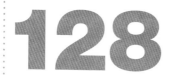

Aloe vera gel is naturally soothing and calming, and the perfect antidote to skin that has been overexposed to the sun. Look for natural products with a high aloe vera content or, even better, 100% aloe vera gel. It will help to reduce redness and ease irritation.

129 GIVE SUNBEDS A WIDE BERTH

Some experts have said that the risk of developing skin cancer from using sunbeds has trebled in the last decade, mostly due to the development of super-powerful tanning beds. Cancer research organizations always advise against the use of sunbeds, especially by young women.

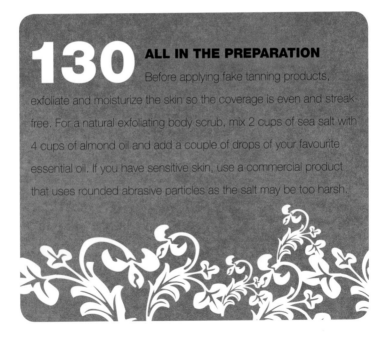

130 ALL IN THE PREPARATION

Before applying fake tanning products, exfoliate and moisturize the skin so the coverage is even and streak-free. For a natural exfoliating body scrub, mix 2 cups of sea salt with 4 cups of almond oil and add a couple of drops of your favourite essential oil. If you have sensitive skin, use a commercial product that uses rounded abrasive particles as the salt may be too harsh.

131

CHOOSE SELF-TAN RATHER THAN A SUNTAN

The sun's rays are one of the main reasons for premature ageing and they also increase the risk of developing skin cancer. The same is true for sunbeds. Research has found that people using sunbeds in their teens and twenties have a 75% increased risk of developing skin cancer. Manufacturers Lavera and Green People both do a natural self-tanning lotion.

132

SAY NO TO TANNING PILLS

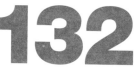

Tanning pills usually contain the pigment canthaxanthin, which is highly dangerous. Although approved for use in food in minimal amounts, in tanning pills it is ingested in high doses and works by changing not only the skin to an orange-brown colour, but also the internal organs. Canthaxanthin has been linked to hepatitis and canthaxanthin retinopathy (yellow deposits in the retina of the eye).

133

WATER IS THE BEST TONER

Avoid expensive, chemical-based toners by rinsing your face water with cold tap water. Some toners contain unnecessarily harsh and astringent chemicals that strip your skin of its natural oils. Cold water will do the same thing toner is designed to do – close up pores and freshen skin after cleansing.

134

BICARBONATE OF SODA FOR HOMEMADE BEAUTY

Bicarbonate of soda (baking soda) is an incredibly versatile natural ingredient. As well as being good for household cleaning, it can also be used for a number of different beauty treatments. Try mixing a small amount with your normal face-cleansing lotion for a homemade exfoliator. Using homemade treatments cuts down on the manufacture, packaging and expense of products, and so reduces your carbon footprint.

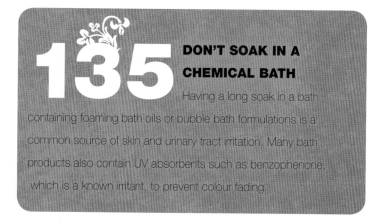

135 DON'T SOAK IN A CHEMICAL BATH

Having a long soak in a bath containing foaming bath oils or bubble bath formulations is a common source of skin and urinary tract irritation. Many bath products also contain UV absorbents such as benzophenone, which is a known irritant, to prevent colour fading.

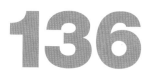

136 BABIES DON'T NEED BUBBLES

It may seem inviting to bathe your little ones in water full of soapy suds but in reality you are simply exposing them to an unnecessary chemical soup. All that's needed to keep infants clean is warm, clean water so avoid the millions of so-called baby-friendly products on the market and keep it simple.

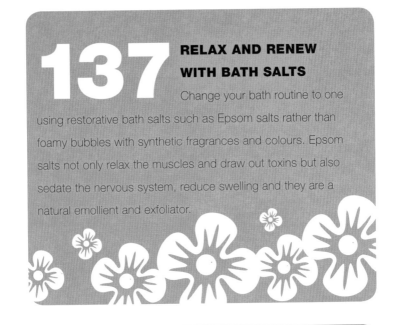

137 RELAX AND RENEW WITH BATH SALTS

Change your bath routine to one using restorative bath salts such as Epsom salts rather than foamy bubbles with synthetic fragrances and colours. Epsom salts not only relax the muscles and draw out toxins but also sedate the nervous system, reduce swelling and they are a natural emollient and exfoliator.

138 MAKE YOUR OWN BATH SALTS

Avoid fragrances and preservatives found in conventional bubble baths and create your own natural bath salts. A good recipe for a tension-relieving bath is to mix Epsom salts with baking soda and a few drops of lavender and marjoram essential oils.

139

MAKE YOUR OWN BATH LOTIONS

Dried thyme and some raw oats make a relaxing and soothing all-natural herbal bath. Place them in a cheesecloth square and either tie it under the tap (faucet) as the water is running or place it directly in the bath. The oatmeal will soften the water.

140

RELAX IN A BATH LIT BY PETROCHEMICAL-FREE CANDLES

Vegetable-based or beeswax candles are better for the environment and better for your health. When lit, normal paraffin candles emit trace amounts of toxins including formaldehyde and petroleum soot. Choose vegetable-based candles such as soy candles perfumed with pure essential oils for a greener alternative.

141

HAVE A SHOWER RATHER THAN A BATH

A bath uses around 170 litres (45 gallons) of water compared with 80 litres (21 gallons) for a five-minute shower. Therefore, switching from your daily bath to a shower can save over 32,000 litres (8,000 gallons) of water a year. Also a shower uses only 40% of the hot water necessary for a bath.

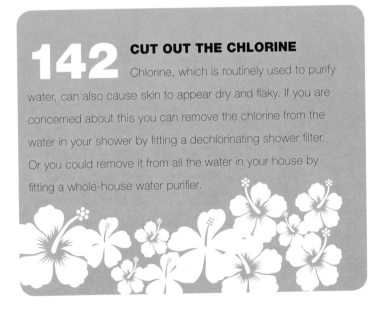

142

CUT OUT THE CHLORINE

Chlorine, which is routinely used to purify water, can also cause skin to appear dry and flaky. If you are concerned about this you can remove the chlorine from the water in your shower by fitting a dechlorinating shower filter. Or you could remove it from all the water in your house by fitting a whole-house water purifier.

143 BUY VEGETABLE OIL SOAPS

Look for vegetable soaps made using the traditional cold-processing method which involves low energy, hand-crafted techniques. These soaps tend to be more suitable for people with sensitive skins and also allergy sufferers as they contain no additives. Caurnie soaps from Scotland also use a double saponification process to produce extra-gentle cleaning products.

144 MAKE YOUR OWN SOAPS

It is not that difficult to create your own home-made soaps and they will be gentler for skin than industrial versions. You will also know exactly what ingredients went into the product. Soap-making kits, widely available from craft stores and online shops, can easily be carried out in the average kitchen. The main ingredients are vegetable oils, caustic soda and essential oils for fragrance.

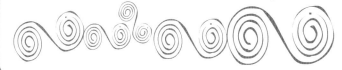

145 CHOOSE SOAP INSTEAD OF DETERGENT

Shampoos, shower gels and bubble baths all rely on detergents, very often the same ones used in heavy industry and cleaning products. Choose soap instead of liquid detergents – it's a natural product made using a fairly low-intensity manufacturing process.

146 DON'T BUY ANTIBACTERIAL SOAP

We are inundated with advertising telling us the best way to get rid of germs from our homes and promoting the use of antibacterial soap in the bathroom. Some studies have found that antibacterial soaps actually contribute to the increase in 'superbugs', and can cause dry skin and hand eczema.

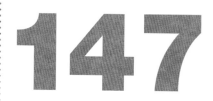

147 LOOK OUT FOR HANDMADE VEGETABLE SOAPS

Vegetable oil and glycerine soaps work as well as any shower gel and come without the cocktail of chemicals in many products. Choose soaps made from coconut, hemp and olive oils – organic, if possible. Handmade soaps are even better as they further reduce the product's environmental impact.

148 DISPOSE OF COTTON BUDS WISELY

Cotton buds (swabs) are one of the worst polluters of our seas, mainly because they are non-biodegradable and yet lots of people flush them down the toilet rather than throwing them out as waste. Research by the Marine Conservation Society in the UK found that cotton buds are the second most common polluter of beaches and seas.

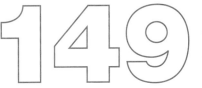

149 BUY ORGANIC COTTON WOOL

Cotton production has a huge environmental impact due to the amount of chemicals used. A recent report found that cotton is responsible for the release of 15% of global insecticides, more than any other single crop. Buy certified organic cotton balls instead.

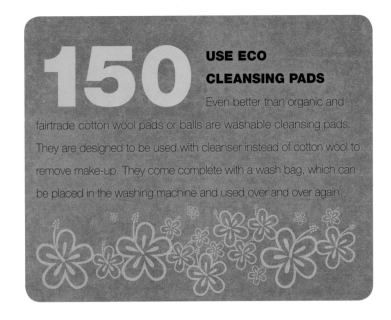

150 USE ECO CLEANSING PADS

Even better than organic and fairtrade cotton wool pads or balls are washable cleansing pads. They are designed to be used with cleanser instead of cotton wool to remove make-up. They come complete with a wash bag, which can be placed in the washing machine and used over and over again.

151

WIPE AWAY WITH WASHABLE WIPES

Instead of relying on disposable baby wipes, some of which contain ingredients such as parabens, which have been linked to cancer, use washable wipes for baby's bottom. As well as avoiding exposure to chemicals you will also reduce the amount of waste you create.

152

GO ORGANIC WITH BABY WIPES

Lots of the mainstream brands of baby wipes contain parabens and propylene glycol, a common ingredient in anti-freeze, so look for certified organic, hypoallergenic and flushable varieties. Alternatively, avoid altogether: a damp cloth or cotton wool dipped in water will do the job just as well.

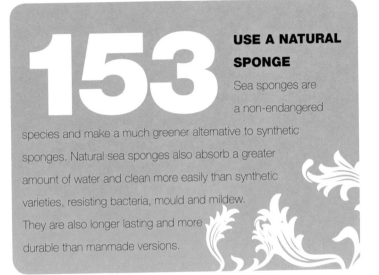

153 USE A NATURAL SPONGE

Sea sponges are a non-endangered species and make a much greener alternative to synthetic sponges. Natural sea sponges also absorb a greater amount of water and clean more easily than synthetic varieties, resisting bacteria, mould and mildew. They are also longer lasting and more durable than manmade versions.

154 LOVE YOUR LOOFAH

Instead of lathering up with a manmade sponge, use a natural loofah, but make sure it has been grown organically and is unbleached. A loofah is a dried plant related to the squash family. Gentle enough to be used every day, it will boost your circulatory system, cleanse and exfoliate your skin, and help prevent cellulite build-up.

155

SOURCE YOUR SPONGES SUSTAINABLY

Natural sea sponges are a greener alternative to synthetic versions, which are generally derived from petrochemicals. However, they are only acceptable if they are sustainably harvested – in the past natural seabed habitats have been disturbed by unsustainable harvesting.

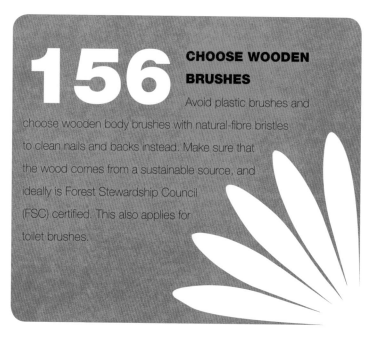

156

CHOOSE WOODEN BRUSHES

Avoid plastic brushes and choose wooden body brushes with natural-fibre bristles to clean nails and backs instead. Make sure that the wood comes from a sustainable source, and ideally is Forest Stewardship Council (FSC) certified. This also applies for toilet brushes.

157

MAKE YOUR BATHROOM PLASTIC-FREE

Swap plastic soap dishes for wooden alternatives and make your bathroom a plastic-free haven. Plastic is derived from petrochemicals and has a major environmental impact during its manufacture and disposal. Stainless steel, which can be recycled, is also a greener option.

158

PROTECT YOURSELF WITH ORGANIC

Avoid the chemicals and dyes in sanitary protection by choosing organic products. The Natracare range of tampons and towels uses 100% organic, non-chlorine bleached and GM-free cotton. They also avoid the unnecessary dyes used to colour the cotton pulls on tampons, which helps to reduce the product's environmental impact.

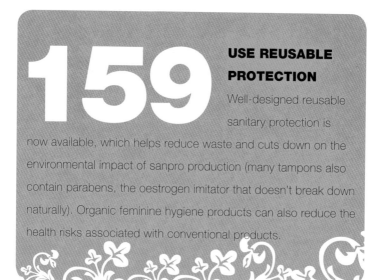

159 USE REUSABLE PROTECTION

Well-designed reusable sanitary protection is now available, which helps reduce waste and cuts down on the environmental impact of sanpro production (many tampons also contain parabens, the oestrogen imitator that doesn't break down naturally). Organic feminine hygiene products can also reduce the health risks associated with conventional products.

160 USE ALL-NATURAL SEA SPONGE TAMPONS

These are a safe, sustainably harvested alternative to conventional tampons and towels. They are completely natural and biodegradable and contain no chemicals, thereby reducing the risk of related diseases such as Toxic Shock Syndrome, which have been connected with standard tampons. As they are reusable sea sponges, they contain no plastic applicators, synthetic fibres or dyes.

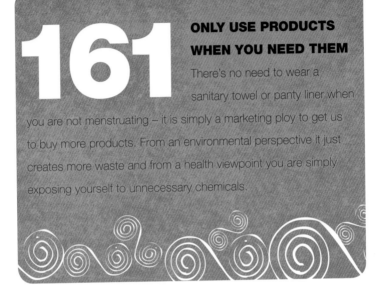

161

ONLY USE PRODUCTS WHEN YOU NEED THEM

There's no need to wear a sanitary towel or panty liner when you are not menstruating – it is simply a marketing ploy to get us to buy more products. From an environmental perspective it just creates more waste and from a health viewpoint you are simply exposing yourself to unnecessary chemicals.

162

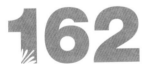

TRY A MOONCUP

A Mooncup is a reusable feminine hygiene product that is gentle on the body, kind to the environment and economical. Made from soft silicone rubber, the Mooncup is worn internally. It can replace tampons and towels, even at night, thereby reducing your exposure to unwanted chemicals.

163 KEEP THE POWDER ON YOUR NOSE

Research has found that women who regularly use talcum powder in their underwear have a 17% higher risk of ovarian cancer than those who did not. Previous studies have suggested that the use of talcum powder might increase the risk of ovarian cancer by as much as 33% over a lifetime.

164 MAKE YOUR OWN TALC

Since talcum powder has been linked to an increased risk of ovarian cancer , it's better to make your own, natural version. A simple body powder can be made by mixing one cup of cornflour (cornstarch) with 10 to 30 drops of essential oil of your choice such as lavender or ylang ylang.

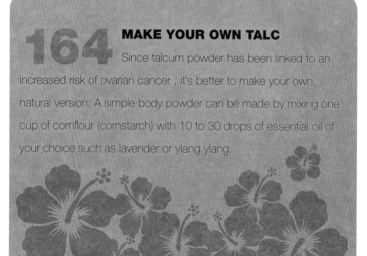

165

DITCH THE AEROSOL FOR A ROLL-ON

Research has found that women who use aerosol deodorant are more likely to have health problems such as headaches and depression than those who don't. The evidence also revealed that using aerosols around young children could adversely affect their health, causing diarrhoea and other symptoms.

166

DON'T SWEAT IT

A natural crystal deodorant will stop bacteria from multiplying and provide protection from sweating while reducing your exposure to chemicals such as parabens, found in many standard deodorant products. Parabens have been linked with breast cancer and hormone disruption, with scientists finding traces of parabens in tissue taken from women with breast cancer.

167 DO SWEAT IT

Much has been written about aluminium's potential to adversely affect our health. Aluminium salts are widely used in antiperspirants because they are very effective at preventing sweating; this in itself is not a great idea because perspiring is an essential way to naturally eliminate toxins from the body. More worrying is the fact that aluminium in antiperspirants has been linked to cancer and found in the breast tissue of women suffering from breast cancer. Use a natural mineral salt or plant extract-based deodorant instead.

168 CHOOSE NATURAL DEODORANTS

Deodorants often contain antibacterial ingredients and fragrance to minimize the odour-producing bacteria created by sweat. However, these ingredients often include triclosan, a known irritant, and parabens. Choose natural deodorants containing essential oils for fragrance, with natural antibacterial properties instead.

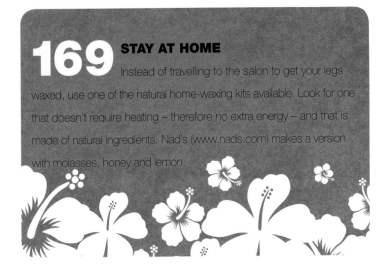

169 STAY AT HOME

Instead of travelling to the salon to get your legs waxed, use one of the natural home-waxing kits available. Look for one that doesn't require heating – therefore no extra energy – and that is made of natural ingredients. Nad's (www.nads.com) makes a version with molasses, honey and lemon.

170 DITCH YOUR DISPOSABLE RAZORS

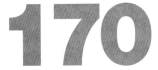

Men and women should avoid using disposable razors that are simply destined for the garbage bin. There's no need to purchase a product that has to be thrown away after a couple of uses – the emissions caused by their production and the waste created is completely avoidable. Invest in a decent razor and simply replace the blades when necessary.

171
GET A CLOSE SHAVE WITH RECYCLED RAZORS

The award-winning Preserve recycled razor is an environmentally friendly alternative to the disposable razor. Made from recycled yogurt pots, the razors have a twin-blade head that can be easily replaced. The handle is made from 100% recycled plastics, 65% of which is recycled yogurt pots. For more information on Preserve-branded products, see Recycline at www.recycline.com.

172
SOLAR SHAVING

Invest in a solar-powered shaver for the ultimate in green shaving. The Sol-Shaver, a solar-powered shaver, has an integrated solar panel and needs to be left out in the sun to charge first. Ideal for travel and camping trips as well as everyday, energy-free shaving, you can charge it on a windowsill, outside in the sun – or even on the dashboard of your car.

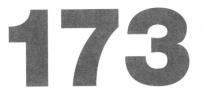

173

TURN ON YOUR MAN

Take advantage of the growing number of natural and organic brands specifically targeting male grooming. The number of paraben-free and SLS (sodium lauryl sulphate)-free shaving foams and gels is rapidly growing so even the greenest men have a wide choice of products. Scoop of Nature is a men-only range of organic skincare (see www.scoopofnature.com).

174

TRY SHAVING SOAP RATHER THAN FOAM

Using a soap to prepare hair for shaving rather than shaving foam will mean less exposure to the solvents and propellants in shaving foam, all of which can cause allergic reactions. Even better, use a vegetable-based shaving oil, which will help to moisturize the skin naturally at the same time.

175 ALOE, ALOE

Aloe vera gel is a great alternative to shaving foams and gels. This is because it has natural anti-inflammatory and skin-softening properties without any added chemicals. You can buy pure aloe gel from most health food stores but why not get your own aloe vera plant?

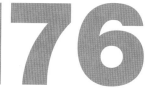

176 CALM SKIN WITH ALOE VERA

Rather than buy an after-shave lotion containing chemicals that may actually irritate newly-shaved skin, use 100% aloe vera gel instead. This is available from health food stores and will soothe and calm the skin without causing any adverse skin reactions.

177

GET THREADING

If you regularly get your eyebrows waxed, try threading for a natural alternative. A traditional Middle Eastern and Asian technique for hair-removal, the specially-trained therapist uses a thin cotton strand, which is twisted and pulled along the skin surface, to lift the hair directly from the follicle. The only material used is the cotton thread and you avoid exposure to the chemicals used during waxing. As it is completely natural, it is suitable for all skin types, and won't result in any irritation or rashes.

178

SOOTHE EYEBROWS WITH HONEY

After plucking your eyebrows apply an astringent such as witch hazel with some cotton wool. Then smooth on a thin layer of honey using your fingers. Leave for a few minutes before rinsing off with warm water. The natural antibacterial properties of honey will soothe and cleanse your brows.

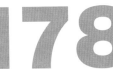

179 SWAP THE CONTACT LENSES FOR GLASSES

Contact lenses have a much greater impact on the environment than spectacles due to their disposable nature and the energy that goes into their manufacture. If you can bear it, swap your lenses for a pair of glasses that you will enjoy wearing, or at least wear your glasses more often to reduce your reliance on contact lenses.

180 AVOID HARSH EYE-WASHES

Eye-wash solutions often contain harsh chemicals. Brighten eyes naturally by using a cold-water wash instead. Then place a hot flannel over closed eyelids and press gently with your fingertips. Alternate this process several times and finish by placing a slice of chilled cucumber over each eye.

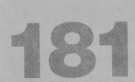

181

CHOOSE YOUR TOOTHPASTE CAREFULLY

Toothpaste is one of the worst culprits when it comes to excessive packaging, with most relying on plastic tubes surrounded by cardboard containers. Look out for brands that use tubes made from biodegradable cellulose, such as Kingfisher, which has a range of natural toothpastes containing ingredients such as lemon, fennel and peppermint.

182

AVOID PUMP-ACTION DISPENSERS

When buying toothpaste avoid the pump-action dispensers. These are really unnecessary and use even more plastic than regular tubes. They cannot be recycled easily and therefore end up on landfill sites where they won't decompose.

183 BRUSH UP WITH BICARBONATE OF SODA

Avoid additive-laden toothpastes by mixing your own using bicarbonate of soda (baking soda), an ingredient which most early toothpastes were based on. It can be mixed with lemon juice to form a toothpaste-like consistency and used in the same way.

184 AVOID ARTIFICIAL COLOURS IN YOUR TOOTHPASTE

Look out for natural, SLS (sodium lauryl sulfate)-free toothpaste without added colours. There's no need for multicoloured stripes when you're brushing your teeth. Look for brands using natural ingredients such as fennel and peppermint, which have natural breath-freshening and antiseptic properties.

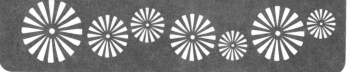

185 FORGET FLUORIDE

There is enough fluoride in the average-sized tube of family toothpaste to endanger the life of a small child if ingested, and in some countries, including the US and Sweden, fluoride toothpastes carry a health warning. In the US this includes the instruction to contact a poison-control centre if more than the amount used for brushing teeth is swallowed. Fluoride has also been linked to allergic-type reactions, diabetes, bone problems and mental impairment.

186 JUST BRUSH, DON'T WHITEN

A report by the Trading Standards Institute in the UK recently reported that 18 out of 20 teeth-whitening products that it tested contained illegal levels of the bleach hydrogen peroxide. High levels of hydrogen peroxide are thought to cause health problems such as chemical burns to the mouth, as well as exacerbating gum disease and heightened sensitivity in teeth.

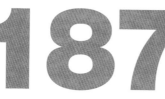

187

REPLACE YOUR HEAD

Reduce plastic waste and landfill impact by using a toothbrush with a replaceable head. Monte Blanco and Smile Brite brands do ranges of replaceable head toothbrushes in various firmnesses for adults and children that are no more expensive than standard brushes and work out cheaper in the long run.

188

TAKE CARE WITH TITANIUM DIOXIDE

Research has shown that many currently fashionable teeth-whitening toothpastes and agents contain titanium dioxide. A suspected carcinogen which can be absorbed into the skin, it is also harmful to the environment and has been found to acidify rivers and seas. It is used both as a pigment and a thickener in many other cosmetic and skincare products.

189

EAT STRAWBERRIES FOR WHITE TEETH

For centuries strawberries have been used to treat discoloured teeth. They can be mashed and applied directly onto teeth to help remove stains caused by red wine or tobacco, providing a healthy natural alternative to chemical teeth-whitening kits that can contain peroxide and titanium dioxide.

190

WASH YOUR MOUTH OUT

There are concerns that conventional mouthwashes may cause an increased risk of throat and mouth cancers. This is because they often contain alcohol, which is drying and changes the acidity of the mouth. Make your own instead by adding a few drops of peppermint oil or sage tincture to water.

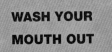

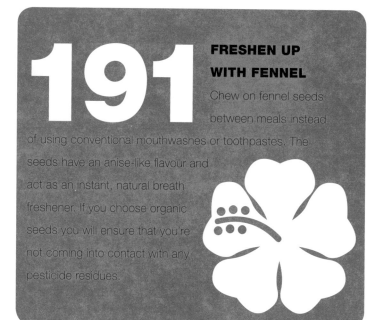

191

FRESHEN UP WITH FENNEL

Chew on fennel seeds between meals instead of using conventional mouthwashes or toothpastes. The seeds have an anise-like flavour and act as an instant, natural breath freshener. If you choose organic seeds you will ensure that you're not coming into contact with any pesticide residues.

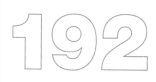

192

SWITCH OFF WHILE YOU BRUSH

This may sound obvious but plenty of people don't do it – turn off the water while you are brushing your teeth. This simple action can save up to 5 litres (8 pints) of water every time you brush!

193 BANISH BAD BREATH WITH A TONGUE SCRAPER

Tongue scrapers have been used in dental hygiene for centuries. They are particularly effective for eliminating bad breath because they dislodge bacteria at the back of the tongue that can be the underlying cause. Using a tongue scraper to freshen breath is a much more natural and environmentally friendly alternative to harsh mouthwashes.

194 USE AN IONIC TOOTHBRUSH

The Soladay ionic toothbrush contains a metal rod made up of a patented semiconductor material. When this is activated by light it produces electrons that help to remove dental plaque without the need for toothpaste, although toothpaste can also be used if you prefer the taste.

195 NATURAL TOOTHBRUSHES

The root of the araak tree (*salvadora persica*) has been traditionally used to clean teeth for centuries in the Middle East. Natural araak toothbrushes, also called sewak or siwak brushes, resemble twigs and contain a number of nutrients that are ideal for maintaining healthy teeth, including vitamin C and minerals. They also have the advantage of not needing toothpaste.

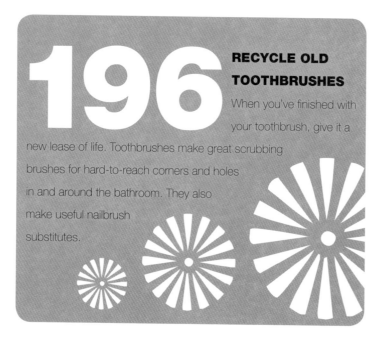

196 RECYCLE OLD TOOTHBRUSHES

When you've finished with your toothbrush, give it a new lease of life. Toothbrushes make great scrubbing brushes for hard-to-reach corners and holes in and around the bathroom. They also make useful nailbrush substitutes.

197 USE SAGE FOR HEALTHY TEETH

Traditionally the herb sage has been used for dental care. It is thought to whiten the enamel of the teeth as well as strengthen the gums. The herb is often included in natural toothpastes and mouthwashes but you can make your own handmade products by mixing sage, fennel and cinnamon essential oils with water.

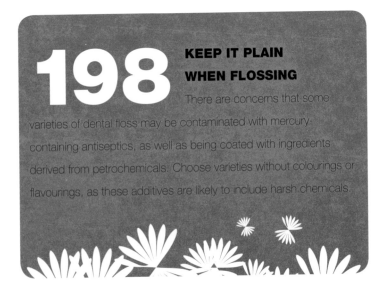

198 KEEP IT PLAIN WHEN FLOSSING

There are concerns that some varieties of dental floss may be contaminated with mercury-containing antiseptics, as well as being coated with ingredients derived from petrochemicals. Choose varieties without colourings or flavourings, as these additives are likely to include harsh chemicals.

199 STRENGTHEN NAILS NATURALLY

Conventional nail-strengthening products often contain formaldehyde, which many people are allergic to and which is also a known carcinogen. Strengthen nails naturally by taking supplements with essential fatty acids and biotin (one of the B vitamins), and by eating enough protein (your nails are made of the natural protein keratin). Keep your nails from drying out and splitting by moisturizing daily.

200 CHOOSE NATURAL NAIL POLISH

Conventional nail varnishes and removers are essentially cocktails of toxic chemicals, such as toluene and colour lakes (colour bases that don't break down in nature), acetone, formaldehyde and phthalates. Look for the BDIH label instead: this is a respected German association for certified natural cosmetics that guarantees a product based on plant oils and herbal and floral extracts from managed cultivation. The products it endorses do not include any organic-synthetic dyes, synthetic fragrances or mineral oil derivatives. Sante Natural Nail Polishes are certified by the BDIH.

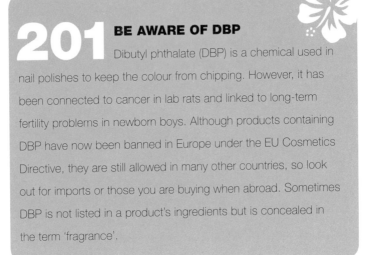

201 BE AWARE OF DBP

Dibutyl phthalate (DBP) is a chemical used in nail polishes to keep the colour from chipping. However, it has been connected to cancer in lab rats and linked to long-term fertility problems in newborn boys. Although products containing DBP have now been banned in Europe under the EU Cosmetics Directive, they are still allowed in many other countries, so look out for imports or those you are buying when abroad. Sometimes DBP is not listed in a product's ingredients but is concealed in the term 'fragrance'.

202 FORGET THE FALSE NAILS

Artificial nails that are not stuck down properly can lead to bacterial or fungal infections, which can in turn cause the loss of a fingernail. Removing artificial nails is also problematic because solvents for artificial nail glue can be extremely toxic – some have been banned in the EU. A report by the University of Toronto revealed that children whose mothers worked in nail salons during pregnancy performed poorly in tests for concentration and language.

203 GO BARE

Instead of using nail polish, protect your nails by rubbing organic almond oil into the nails and cuticles to strengthen them. Clean discoloured nails by scrubbing them with a slice of lemon, which will get rid of stains, and gently buff for all-natural shine.

204 PAINT JOB

Because nail colours can contain powerful chemicals such as formaldehyde, solvents and allergens that may irritate the skin, protect your cuticles with a vegetable oil before you paint your nails. Dab on plain organic olive or almond oil around the nail bed, or alternatively look for a natural cuticle cream containing such ingredients as shea butter, seabuckthorn berry extract and essential oils.

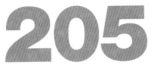

205 BE ANIMAL-FRIENDLY

Vegetarians and vegans should be aware that make-up often contains a number of different animal ingredients. These include stearic acid and glycerin, sorbitan or octyl stearate, cochineal/carmine and silk. Vegans should also look out for beeswax, honey and lanolin. Animal-friendly brands include Dr Hauschka and The Body Shop.

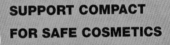

206 SUPPORT COMPACT FOR SAFE COSMETICS

Choose cosmetics brands where the manufacturers have signed up to the Compact for Safe Cosmetics campaign, which is run by the US-based Environmental Working Group. Each company pledges not to use chemicals that may cause cancer or birth defects in their products and to replace any hazardous materials with safer alternatives. For more information on the companies who partake in the campaign, visit www.safecosmetics.org/companies.

207 MAKE-UP WITH MINERALS

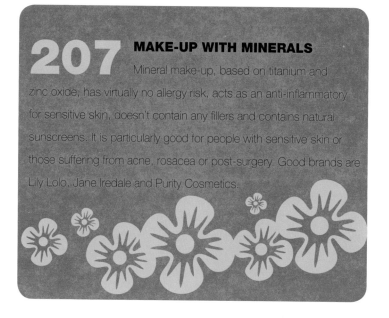

Mineral make-up, based on titanium and zinc oxide, has virtually no allergy risk, acts as an anti-inflammatory for sensitive skin, doesn't contain any fillers and contains natural sunscreens. It is particularly good for people with sensitive skin or those suffering from acne, rosacea or post-surgery. Good brands are Lily Lolo, Jane Iredale and Purity Cosmetics.

208 OPEN YOUR EYES TO NATURAL MASCARA

Many people react badly to mascara, and this is usually due to the chemicals and preservatives, including parabens, used in manufacture. The chemicals employed as drying agents can cause itchy, watery eyes, redness and swelling. Invest in a natural or organic mascara that is free from petrochemicals and alcohol.

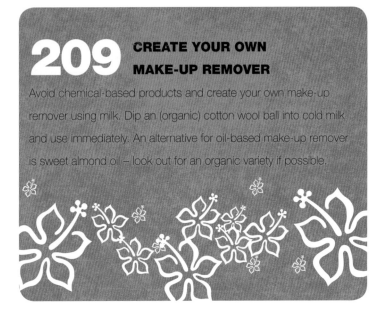

209 CREATE YOUR OWN MAKE-UP REMOVER

Avoid chemical-based products and create your own make-up remover using milk. Dip an (organic) cotton wool ball into cold milk and use immediately. An alternative for oil-based make-up remover is sweet almond oil – look out for an organic variety if possible.

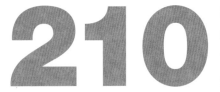

210 BARE-FACED CHEEK

Try going make-up free for one or two days a week to give your skin a chance to recover and breathe, especially if you are a regular wearer of pore-blocking cosmetics like foundation. Being bare-faced will also help reduce your exposure to chemicals.

211 REMOVE MAKE-UP WITH A COMBINED CLEANSER

Instead of buying two different products, one for make-up removal and one for skin-cleansing, choose a product that is formulated to do both jobs. Choose a gentle, plant-based product that won't irritate your eyes when taking off mascara, but which will moisturize your skin as well as cleaning it.

212 CHOOSE LESS VIVID COLOURS FOR YOUR MAKE-UP

They are pretty but at what cost? A general rule of thumb when it comes to cosmetics is that the brighter the colour of a particular cosmetic, the more toxic it is likely to be. By choosing more neutral shades you will be helping to reduce demand for the most environmentally unfriendly pigments.

213

KEEP AN EYE ON INGREDIENTS

Many mainstream eyeshadows contain coal tar, albeit in tiny amounts. Lipstick is another product that sometimes holds high levels of artificial colourings made from coal-tar derivatives. Coal tar has been linked to cancer and has been found to cause allergic reactions in some people.

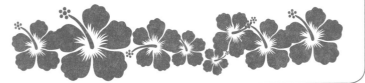

214

DON'T FORGET YOUR BEDTIME RITUAL

It is important to remove all traces of make-up before you go to sleep, so never miss out on this step. Mascara left on the eyes can flake into the eye and scratch the cornea, cause irritation or infection. Leaving make-up such as foundation on overnight can clog pores and dehydrate the skin.

215 LOOK CLOSELY AT YOUR LIPSTICK

The average woman will consume 1 kg (2 lb) of lipstick in her lifetime. Not a pleasant thought when you consider that most lipsticks contain synthetic dyes and fragrances, petroleum derivatives, preservatives such as butylated hydroxyanisole (BHT) and even lead. Choose lipsticks and glosses made using natural products such as beeswax and plant oils, which you won't mind eating.

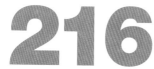

216 GET ORGANICALLY LIPPY

The first certified organic lipstick in the UK was launched by Green People in 2006, following organic lipsticks by Nvey Eco and Hemp Organics in the US and Australia. Organic lippy is made using plant-based oils such as coconut and jojoba rather than petroleum-based ingredients. Green People's version contains fairly traded cupuaçu butter from the Brazilian Amazonian basin. See www.greenpeople.co.uk and www.econveybeauty.com for product information.

217 CRANBERRY DIY LIPSTICK

Avoid the petrochemicals and other ingredients found in lipsticks such as castor oil and even lead by making your own. Mix almond oil with ten fresh cranberries and a teaspoon of honey. Heat in a microwave for a couple of minutes. Mash the berries and then strain through a fine sieve before allowing it to cool.

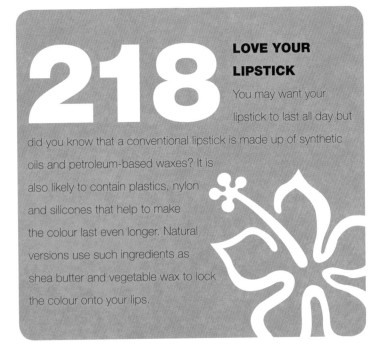

218 LOVE YOUR LIPSTICK

You may want your lipstick to last all day but did you know that a conventional lipstick is made up of synthetic oils and petroleum-based waxes? It is also likely to contain plastics, nylon and silicones that help to make the colour last even longer. Natural versions use such ingredients as shea butter and vegetable wax to lock the colour onto your lips.

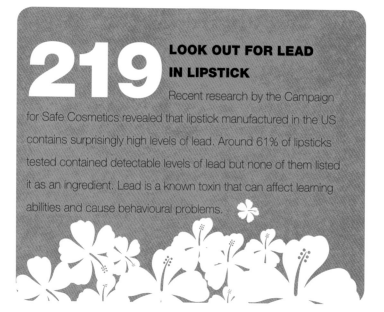

219

LOOK OUT FOR LEAD IN LIPSTICK

Recent research by the Campaign for Safe Cosmetics revealed that lipstick manufactured in the US contains surprisingly high levels of lead. Around 61% of lipsticks tested contained detectable levels of lead but none of them listed it as an ingredient. Lead is a known toxin that can affect learning abilities and cause behavioural problems.

220

MISS A WASH (OR TWO)

If you usually wash your hair every day, try leaving it for two or three days instead. Over-washing hair with chemical-based shampoos and conditioners can strip it of its natural oils. Once you have got used to the new regime you will probably find that your hair looks better and can go even longer between washes.

221 KEY CHEMICALS FOR ASTHMA SUFFERERS TO AVOID

There is increasing evidence that the following ingredients, often found in haircare products, have been linked to asthma in hairdressers. They are: ammonium persulfate, potassium persulfate and sodium persulfate. Asthma sufferers should try to avoid them.

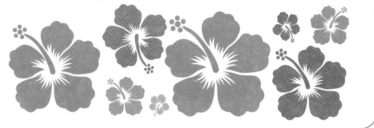

222 BEAT DANDRUFF NATURALLY

Dandruff is an embarrassing problem that sufferers would like to get rid of quickly. Although conventional anti-dandruff shampoos are often effective, they also contain chemicals such as coal tar, which has been linked to cancer. Use a natural shampoo and supplement with essential fatty acids (EFAs) to boost your skin internally instead.

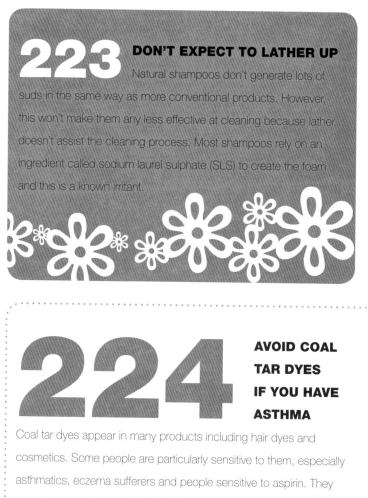

223 DON'T EXPECT TO LATHER UP

Natural shampoos don't generate lots of suds in the same way as more conventional products. However, this won't make them any less effective at cleaning because lather doesn't assist the cleaning process. Most shampoos rely on an ingredient called sodium laurel sulphate (SLS) to create the foam and this is a known irritant.

224 AVOID COAL TAR DYES IF YOU HAVE ASTHMA

Coal tar dyes appear in many products including hair dyes and cosmetics. Some people are particularly sensitive to them, especially asthmatics, eczema sufferers and people sensitive to aspirin. They can also cause hyperactivity in children and severe headaches.

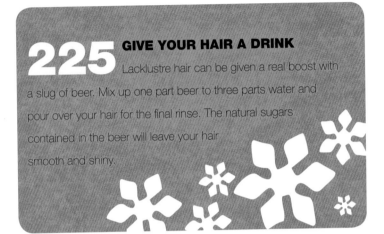

225 GIVE YOUR HAIR A DRINK

Lacklustre hair can be given a real boost with a slug of beer. Mix up one part beer to three parts water and pour over your hair for the final rinse. The natural sugars contained in the beer will leave your hair smooth and shiny.

226 LOOK AFTER YOUR LASHES

Never use permanent hair dyes to colour eyebrows or eyelashes. The chemicals found in these products can cause an allergic reaction or even blindness. Avoid home tinting kits completely and go to a salon if you really can't bear to go 'au naturel'.

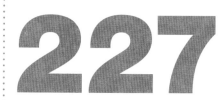

227

NATURAL WAYS TO COMBAT HAIR LOSS

Increasing the amount of protein-rich foods such as eggs, fish and tofu is one way to combat hair loss. Another is to take regular exercise, which will help boost circulation and increase blood flow to the scalp. Massaging your scalp also encourages the blood supply to stimulate hair growth.

228

WASH THOSE CHEMICALS OUT OF YOUR HAIR

Conventional shampoos use the same detergents found in everything from cleaning products to shower gels. One of the health concerns about shampoo is that some of the common ingredients can break down into formaldehyde during storage. Formaldehyde is a known irritant that has been linked to cancer.

229 USE NATURAL HAIR DYES

Mainstream hair dyes use strong chemicals such as ammonia and have been linked to health problems including scalp irritation, facial swelling and even cancer. Choose natural dyes made with vegetable ingredients instead. These are still able to lighten hair by a couple of shades but without the potential side effects caused by harsher dyes and bleaches.

230 THINK BEFORE YOU DYE

Research studies have revealed that hair dyes pose an increased risk of cancer. One such study found that individuals who had worked for ten years or more as a hair stylist could have a risk of bladder cancer, which is five times greater than the general population.

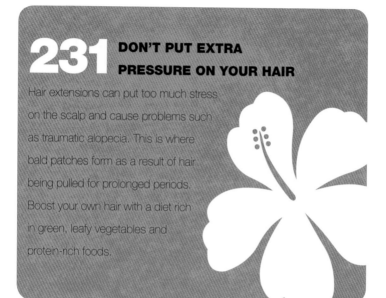

231 DON'T PUT EXTRA PRESSURE ON YOUR HAIR

Hair extensions can put too much stress on the scalp and cause problems such as traumatic alopecia. This is where bald patches form as a result of hair being pulled for prolonged periods. Boost your own hair with a diet rich in green, leafy vegetables and protein-rich foods.

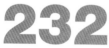

232 HAIR TO DYE FOR

Many people have allergic reactions to hair dye, ranging from tingling of the scalp and general discomfort to facial dermatitis and even facial swelling. Para-phenylenediamine (PPD), one of the ingredients that can trigger allergic reactions, is still found in the majority of mainstream hair dyes despite being banned in Germany, France and Sweden.

233 EMBRACE GREASY HAIR

Give dry hair a natural conditioning treatment with olive oil. The oil helps repair split ends and improves the texture and appearance of parched hair. Heat the oil first in a cup placed in a pan of hot water. Then massage it into your hair and scalp and cover with a shower or swimming cap. Leave for 30 minutes before washing out with a gentle shampoo. Try this treatment once a week to give hair a natural boost or to remedy a dry, itchy scalp.

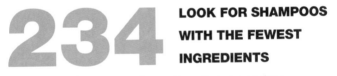

234 LOOK FOR SHAMPOOS WITH THE FEWEST INGREDIENTS

Detergents in shampoo can be problematic because they may break down into formaldehyde during storage. When formaldehyde-forming agents mix with other ingredients they can form nitrosamines, which are linked to cancer. Avoid this cocktail effect by choosing formulas containing minimal ingredients.

235 HOLD THE HAIRSPRAY

Conventional hairsprays coat the hair with a plastic film to hold it in place. Many hairsprays contain phthalates, hormone-disrupting chemicals which have been linked with a number of health scares including birth defects. Choose hairspray made with natural ingredients in pump action rather than aerosol dispensers.

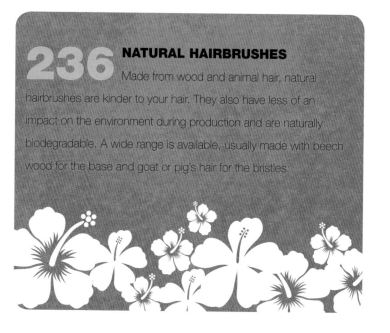

236 NATURAL HAIRBRUSHES

Made from wood and animal hair, natural hairbrushes are kinder to your hair. They also have less of an impact on the environment during production and are naturally biodegradable. A wide range is available, usually made with beech wood for the base and goat or pig's hair for the bristles.

237 DON'T HAVE A SHOWER JUST TO WASH YOUR HAIR

Water is a precious resource and one way to save a considerable amount of it is not to have a bath or shower simply to wash your hair. Use a hand-held shower attachment instead and turn the water off while you apply the shampoo and conditioner.

238 BE CAUTIOUS OF ADDED INGREDIENTS

Hair conditioner may be effective in many ways but it cannot magically repair damaged hair. Neither can it make hair more healthy by adding proteins, vitamins, amino acids or other ingredients. Give your hair a boost with a homemade mixture of fresh rosemary and mint with cider vinegar.

239

UNPLUG THE STRAIGHTENERS

Repeated use of hair straighteners can actually damage your hair, especially if it is fine. From an environmental perspective there is also the consideration of the energy used in their manufacture and during their use. Try to eliminate or reduce your reliance on hair straighteners, tongs, blowdryers and other electric devices to reduce your carbon footprint and save the health of your hair.

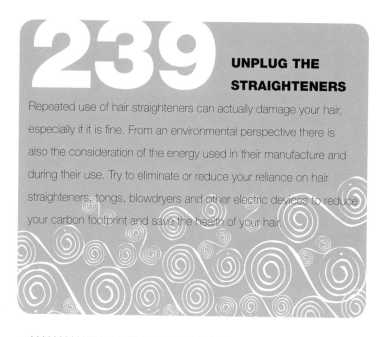

240

DON'T BUY INTO PACKAGING

Research has revealed that as much as 50% of the cost of a bottle of perfume can be accounted for by packaging and advertising. Some companies offer a refill service where you can take in old bottles and get them refilled, cutting back on waste and packaging.

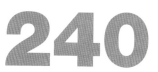

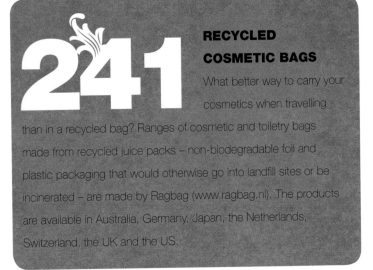

241 RECYCLED COSMETIC BAGS

What better way to carry your cosmetics when travelling than in a recycled bag? Ranges of cosmetic and toiletry bags made from recycled juice packs – non-biodegradable foil and plastic packaging that would otherwise go into landfill sites or be incinerated – are made by Ragbag (www.ragbag.nl). The products are available in Australia, Germany, Japan, the Netherlands, Switzerland, the UK and the US.

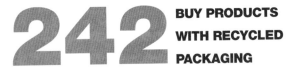

242 BUY PRODUCTS WITH RECYCLED PACKAGING

Packaging is one of the things used to sell cosmetics and beauty products but it is unnecessary and adds to the growing global waste problem. Look for products that use recycled cardboard packaging such as those made by Living Nature and Lavera.

243 BUY GLASS BOTTLES NOT PLASTIC

Packaging will contribute a great deal to the environmental impact of all beauty and bodycare products. Therefore, where possible buy products packaged in glass bottles rather than plastic as these are easier to recycle. Good examples of this include deodorants from Pitrok and Urtekram.

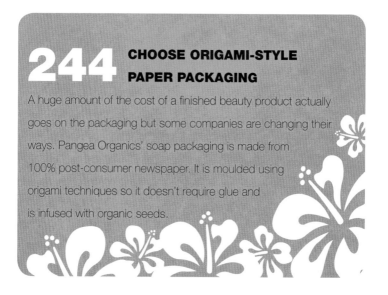

244 CHOOSE ORIGAMI-STYLE PAPER PACKAGING

A huge amount of the cost of a finished beauty product actually goes on the packaging but some companies are changing their ways. Pangea Organics' soap packaging is made from 100% post-consumer newspaper. It is moulded using origami techniques so it doesn't require glue and is infused with organic seeds.

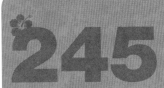

245 BUY IN BULK

It may not be the most glamorous option but try to buy products in the largest size available in order to cut back on packaging. You can then decant into a more convenient, smaller container at home. However, remember to check the shelf-life: you don't want to be left with products past the 'best before' date.

246 TRAVEL LIGHT

Don't buy travel-sized versions of bodycare products when you are going on holiday. These containers are generally thrown away after use and end up on landfill. Instead, use your own small containers to decant your shampoo and shower gel, which can be rinsed out and re-used on your next trip.

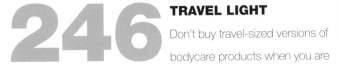

247

AVOID PVC PACKAGING

Aside from the waste issue created by cosmetic packaging there are also health concerns. The manufacturing process of PVC is known to release cancer-causing dioxins into the environment. There are also concerns that chemicals, such as phthalates, may leach out of the plastic container into the product.

248

CUT BACK ON PACKAGING

A number of manufacturers are developing products that require little packaging, such as Lush's solid shampoo bar. Other ways to reduce waste from packaging include recycling schemes such as that offered by The Body Shop.

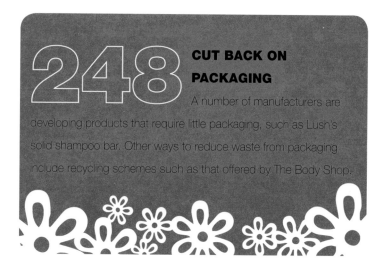

249

USE RECYCLED FACIAL TISSUES

Around 3.2% of the world's commercial timber production goes into the manufacture of tissue products and Greenpeace estimates that an area of ancient forest the size of a football pitch disappears every two seconds in order to feed the demand for paper production. Buying recycled products helps to reduce illegal logging.

250

BUY RECYCLED PRODUCTS

Look out for cosmetics and skincare brands that only use recycled packaging for their products. REN, the skincare company, is one which also uses recycled cartons and filling material for delivering its products. It operates a take-back recycling scheme for its customers, where they will recycle empty bottles sent back to them.

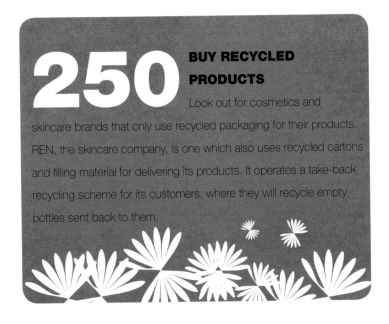